The Complete Cookbook 2021

Your Complete Guide With 100 Easy and Quick Recipes to Living the Keto Lifestyle

Elena Baker

© **Copyright 2021 - All rights reserved.**

The content contained within this book may not be reproduced, duplicated or transmitted without direct written permission from the author or the publisher.

Under no circumstances will any blame or legal responsibility be held against the publisher, or author, for any damages, reparation, or monetary loss due to the information contained within this book. Either directly or indirectly.

Legal Notice:

This book is copyright protected. This book is only for personal use. You cannot amend, distribute, sell, use, quote or paraphrase any part, or the content within this book, without the consent of the author or publisher.

Disclaimer Notice:

Please note the information contained within this document is for educational and entertainment purposes only. All effort has been executed to present accurate, up to date, and reliable, complete information. No warranties of any kind are declared or implied. Readers acknowledge that the author is not engaging in the rendering of legal, financial, medical or professional advice. The content within this book has been derived from various sources. Please consult a licensed professional before attempting any techniques outlined in this book.

By reading this document, the reader agrees that under no circumstances is the author responsible for any losses, direct or indirect, which are incurred as a result of the use of information contained within this document, including, but not limited to, — errors, omissions, or inaccuracies.

TABLE OF CONTENTS

SMOOTHIES & BREAKFAST RECIPES 9
CreamyRaspberrySmoothie 9
Energy Booster Breakfast Smoothie 10
Blackberry Smoothie 11
Choco Sunflower Butter Smoothie 12
CheeseBlueberrySmoothie 13
PORK, BEEF & LAMB RECIPES 14
Juicy & TenderBaked Pork Chops 15
SEAFOOD & FISH RECIPES 17
Delicious Seafood Dip 17
Spinach Shrimp Alfredo 19
Shrimp Scampi 20
MEATLESS MEALS 22
Mexican Cauliflower Rice 22
Balsamic ZucchiniNoodles 24
Cauliflower Broccoli Rice 25
SOUPS, STEWS & SALADS 27
Broccoli Cheese Soup 27
Hearty Cabbage Beef Soup 29
Tasty Taco Soup 31
BRUNCH & DINNER 32
Olive Cheese Omelet 32
Cheese Almond Pancakes 34
DESSERTS & DRINKS 35
Cinnamon AlmondBalls 35
Choco Frosty 36
Cheesecake Fat Bombs 37
BREAKFAST RECIPES 38
Cheesy Ham Souffle 38

Browned Butter Pumpkin Latte 40

Cauliflower Toast with Avocado 41

Breakfast Cheesy Sausage 43

APPETIZERS AND DESSERTS 44

Caprese Snack 44

Almond Flour Crackers 45

Hamburger Patties 47

Buttery Beef Curry 48

Cheesy Beef 49

Beef Quiche 50

Chili Beef 51

SEAFOOD RECIPES 52

Garlic Butter Salmon 52

Tuscan Butter Salmon 54

Mahi Mahi Stew 56

VEGAN & VEGETARIAN 57

Browned Butter Cauliflower Mash 57

Cauliflower Gratin 59

CHICKEN AND POULTRY RECIPES 61

Turkey with Cream Cheese Sauce 61

Keto Pesto Chicken Casserole 62

BREAKFAST RECIPES 63

Cauliflower Zucchini Fritters 63

Flax Almond Muffins 65

Fresh Berries with Cream 67

Chia Flaxseed Waffles 68

Cinnamon Noatmeal 70

Herb Spaghetti Squash 71

Delicious Cabbage Steaks 72

Mexican Cauliflower Rice 73

Asparagus Mash	75
Creamy Squash Soup	76
Spinach with Coconut Milk	77
DINNER RECIPES	78
Roasted Squash	78
Lemon Garlic Mushrooms	79
Almond Green Beans	80
Fried Okra	81
Lemon Mousse	82
BREAKFAST RECIPES	83
Almond Butter Shake	83
Bacon & Egg Fat Bomb	84
Avocado Chicken Salad	86
Burger Cabbage Stir Fry	88
SNACK RECIPES	89
Bacon Wrapped Avocado	89
DINNER RECIPES	91
Beef & Broccoli Stir fry	91
Beef Kheema Meatloaf	93
UNUSUAL DDELICIOUS MEAL RECIPES	95
Blackberry Clafoutis Tarts	95
Calamari Salad	98
Pumpkin Bars	100
Flavors Pumpkin Bars	102
Coconut Lemon Bars	103
CAKE	105
Beginner:Delicious Ricotta Cake	105
Chocó Coconut Cake	107
Fudgy Chocolate Cake	109
Cinnamon Almond Cake	110
Intermediate: Lemon Cake	112

CANDY: BEGINNER	113
Strawberry Candy	113
Blackberry Candy	114
COOKIES: BEGINNER	115
Almond Butter Cookies	115
Crunchy Shortbread Cookies	116
Raspberry Yogurt	117
Coconut ButterPopsicle	118
Raspberry Sorbet	119
Strawberry Yogurt	120
Beginners:SimmeredGarlic Bread	121
Basil Pesto Bread	123
Broken Black PepperBread	124
PennsylvaniaDutchPotato and Bread Filling	126
LUNCH RECIPES	128
Beginners: Low-Carb Cream Cheese Rolls	128
Homemade Sesame Breadsticks	130
Herb Bread	131
Almond Keto Bread	132
SNACKS RECIPES	133
Beginners: Breadwith zucchini and walnuts	133
Garlic bread	135
Sesame bread	136
Focaccia	137
THE KETO LUNCH	138
Monday: Lunch: Keto Meatballs	138
Tuesday:Lunch:MasonJar Salad	140
Wednesday: Lunch: The Smoked Salmon Special	141
KETO AT DINNER	142
Monday: Dinner: Beefshort ribs in a slow cooker	142

SMOOTHIES & BREAKFAST

Creamy Raspberry Smoothie

Preparation Time: 5 minutes Cooking Time: 5 minutes

Serve: 2

Ingredients:

- 1 cup unsweetened almond milk
- 1/2 tsp vanilla
- 1 tbsp cream cheese, softened
- 2 tbsp swerve
- 1/4 cup fresh raspberries
- 4 tbsp heavy cream
- 1 cup ice

Directions:

1. Add all ingredients into the blender and blend until smooth and creamy.
2. Serve and enjoy.

Nutritional Value (Amount per Serving):

Calories 157

Fat 14.7 g

Carbohydrates 4.9 g

Sugar 0.9 g

Protein 1.7 g

Cholesterol 47 mg

Energy Booster Breakfast Smoothie

Preparation Time: 5 minutes Cooking Time: 5 minutes

Serve: 1

Ingredients:

- 1 cup unsweetened almond milk
- 1/2 cup ice
- 1 1/2 tsp maca powder
- 1 tbsp almond butter
- 1 tbsp MCT oil

Directions:

1. Add all ingredients into the blender and blend until smooth.
2. Serve and enjoy.

Nutritional Value (Amount per Serving):

Calories 248

Fat 26.5 g

Carbohydrates 4.5 g

Sugar 1.2 g

Protein 4.9 g

Cholesterol 0 mg

Blackberry Smoothie

Preparation Time: 5 minutes Cooking Time: 5 minutes

Serve: 2

Ingredients:

- 1 cup unsweetened almond milk
- 1/2 cup ice
- 1/2 tsp vanilla
- 1 tsp erythritol
- 2 oz cream cheese, softened
- 4 tbsp heavy whipping cream
- 2 oz fresh blackberries

Directions:

1. Add all ingredients into the blender and blend until smooth.
2. Serve and enjoy.

Nutritional Value (Amount per Serving):

Calories 238

Fat 22.9 g

Carbohydrates 5.9 g

Sugar 4.1 g

Protein 3.7 g

Cholesterol 72 mg

Choco Sunflower Butter Smoothie

Preparation Time: 5 minutes Cooking Time: 5 minutes Serve: 1

Ingredients:

- 1/3 cup unsweetened coconut milk
- 1/4 cup ice
- 1/2 tsp vanilla
- 1 tsp unsweetened cocoa powder
- 2/3 cup water
- 2 tbsp sunflower seed butter

Directions:

- Add all ingredients into the blender and blend until smooth.
- Serve and enjoy.

Nutritional Value (Amount per Serving):

Calories 379

Fat 34.6 g

Carbohydrates 13 g

Sugar 3 g

Protein 8.5 g

Cholesterol 0 mg

Cheese Blueberry Smoothie

Preparation Time: 5 minutes Cooking Time: 5 minutes Serve: 1

Ingredients:

- 1 cup unsweetened almond milk
- 1/2 cup ice
- 1/4 tsp vanilla
- 5 drops liquid stevia
- 1 scoop vanilla protein powder
- 1/3 cup blueberries
- 2 oz cream cheese

Directions:

1. Add all ingredients into the blender and blend until smooth.
2. Serve and enjoy.

Nutritional Value (Amount per Serving):

Calories 380

Fat 23.5 g

Carbohydrates 6.1 g

Sugar 5.3 g

Protein 32.7 g

Cholesterol 64 mg

PORK, BEEF & LAMB RECIPES

Pan Fry Pork Chops Preparation Time: 10 minutes Cooking Time: 8 minutes

Serve: 4

Ingredients:

- 4 pork chops, boneless
- 2 tbsp olive oil
- 1/4 tsp onion powder
- 1/4 tsp garlic powder
- 1/4 tsp pepper
- Salt

Directions:

Heat oil in cast iron skillet over high heat.

1. Season pork chops with garlic powder, onion powder, pepper, and salt.
2. Sear pork chops in hot oil about 3-4 minutes on each side.
3. Serve and enjoy.

Nutritional Value (Amount per Serving):

Calories 317
Fat 26 g
Carbohydrates 0.3 g
Sugar 0.1 g
Protein 18 g
Cholesterol 69 mg

Juicy & Tender Baked Pork Chops

Preparation Time: 10 minutes Cooking Time: 35 minutes Serve: 4

Ingredients:

- 4 pork chops, boneless
- 2 tbsp olive oil
- ½ tsp Italian seasoning
- ½ tsp paprika
- ½ tsp garlic powder
- ¼ tsp pepper
- ½ tsp sea salt

Directions:

1. Preheat the oven to 375 F.
2. In a small bowl, mix together garlic powder, paprika, Italian seasoning, pepper, and salt.
3. Brush pork chops with oil and rub with garlic powder mixture.
4. Place pork chops onto a baking tray and bake in preheated oven for 30-35 minutes.
5. Serve and enjoy.

Nutritional Value (Amount per Serving):

Calories 320

Fat 27 g

Carbohydrates 0.5 g

Sugar 0.2 g

Protein 18 g

Cholesterol 69 mg

SEAFOOD & FISH RECIPES

Delicious Seafood Dip

Preparation Time: 10 minutes Cooking Time: 30 minutes

Serve: 16

Ingredients:

- 1/2 lb shrimp, cooked
- 4 oz can green chilies
- 2 cups pepper jack cheese
- 4 oz cream cheese
- 1/2 tsp old bay seasoning
- 2 garlic cloves, minced
- 1/2 cup spinach, minced
- 1/2 cup onion, minced
- 2 tbsp butter
- 4 oz crab meat

Directions:

1. Preheat the oven to 425 F.
2. Melt butter in a pan over medium heat.
3. Add garlic, old bay seasoning, spinach, crab meat, chilies, and shrimp and cook for 4-5 minutes.
4. Add 1 cup pepper jack cheese and cream cheese.

5. Top with remaining cheese and bake for 20 minutes.
6. Serve and enjoy.

Nutritional Value (Amount per Serving):

Calories 63

Fat 4 g

Carbohydrates 1 g

Sugar 0.2 g

Protein 5 g

Cholesterol 45 mg

Spinach Shrimp Alfredo

Preparation Time: 10 minutes Cooking Time: 15 minutes

Serve: 2

Ingredients:

- 1/2 lb shrimp, deveined
- 2 garlic cloves, minced
- 2 tbsp onion, chopped
- 1 cup fresh spinach, chopped
- 1/2 cup heavy cream
- 1 tbsp butter
- Pepper
- Salt

Directions:

1. Melt butter in a pan over medium heat.
2. Add onion, garlic and shrimp in the pan and sauté for 3 minutes.
3. Add remaining ingredients and simmer for 7 minutes or until cooked.
4. Serve and enjoy.

Nutritional Value (Amount per Serving):

Calories 300

Fat 19 g

Carbohydrates 5 g

Sugar 0.5 g

Protein 27 g

Cholesterol 295 mg

Shrimp Scampi

Preparation Time: 10 minutes Cooking Time: 10 minutes

Serve: 4

Ingredients:

- 1 lb shrimp
- 1/4 tsp red pepper flakes
- 1 tbsp fresh lemon juice
- 1/4 cup butter
- 1/2 cup chicken broth
- 2 garlic cloves, minced
- 1 shallot, sliced
- 3 tbsp olive oil
- 3 tbsp parsley, chopped
- Pepper
- Salt

Directions:

1. Heat oil in a pan over medium heat.
2. Add garlic and shallots and cook for 3 minutes.
3. Add broth, lemon juice, and butter and cook for 5 minutes.
4. Add red pepper flakes, parsley, pepper, and salt. Stir.
5. Add shrimp and cook for 3 minutes.
6. Serve and enjoy.

Nutritional Value (Amount per Serving):

Calories 336

Fat 24 g

Carbohydrates 3 g

Sugar 0.2 g

Protein 26 g

Cholesterol 269 mg

MEATLESS MEALS

Mexican Cauliflower Rice

Preparation Time: 10 minutes Cooking Time: 10 minutes Serve: 3

Ingredients:

- 1 large cauliflower head, cut into florets
- 2 garlic cloves, minced
- 1 onion, diced
- 1 tbsp olive oil
- 1/4 cup vegetable broth
- 3 tbsp tomato paste
- 1/2 tsp cumin
- 1 tsp salt

Directions:

1. Add cauliflower in food processor and process until it looks like rice.
2. Heat oil in a pan over medium heat.
3. Add onion and garlic and sauté for 3 minutes.
4. Add cauliflower rice, cumin, and salt and stir well.
5. Add broth and tomato paste and stir until well combined.

6. Serve and enjoy.

Nutritional Value (Amount per Serving):

Calories 90

Fat 5 g

Carbohydrates 10 g

Sugar 4 g

Protein 3 g

Cholesterol 0 mg

Balsamic Zucchini Noodles

Preparation Time: 10 minutes Cooking Time: 15 minutes Serve: 4

Ingredients:

- 4 zucchinis, spiralized using a slicer
- 1 1/2 tbsp balsamic vinegar
- 1/4 cup fresh basil leaves, chopped
- 4 mozzarella balls, quartered
- 1 1/2 cups cherry tomatoes, halved
- 2 tbsp olive oil
- Pepper
- Salt

Directions:

1. Add zucchini noodles in a bowl and season with pepper and salt. Set aside for 10 minutes.
2. Add mozzarella, tomatoes, and basil and toss well.
3. Drizzle with oil and balsamic vinegar.
4. Serve and enjoy.

Nutritional Value (Amount per Serving):

Calories 222

Fat 15 g

Carbohydrates 10 g

Sugar 5.8 g

Protein 9.5 g

Cholesterol 13 mg

Cauliflower Broccoli Rice

Preparation Time: 10 minutes Cooking Time: 8 minutes Serve: 4

Ingredients:

- 1 cup broccoli, process into rice
- 3 cups cauliflower rice
- 1/4 cup mascarpone cheese
- 1/2 cup parmesan cheese, shredded
- 1/8 tsp ground cinnamon
- ¼ tsp garlic powder
- ¼ tsp onion powder
- 1/4 tsp pepper
- 1 tbsp butter, melted
- 1/2 tsp salt

Directions:

1. In a heat-safe bowl, mix together cauliflower, nutmeg, garlic powder, onion powder, butter, broccoli, pepper, and salt and microwave for 4 minutes.
2. Stir well and microwave for 2 minutes more.
3. Add cheese and microwave for 2 minutes.
4. Add mascarpone cheese and stir until it looks creamy.
5. Serve and enjoy.

Nutritional Value (Amount per Serving):

Calories 135

Fat 10 g

Carbohydrates 6 g

Sugar 2 g

Protein 8 g

Cholesterol 30 mg

SOUPS, STEWS & SALADS

Broccoli Cheese Soup

Preparation Time: 10 minutes Cooking Time: 2 hours 30 minutes

Serve: 4

Ingredients:

- 5 cups broccoli florets
- 2 cups cheddar cheese, shredded
- 1/2 cup mozzarella cheese, shredded
- 4 tbsp cream cheese
- 3 tbsp butter
- ½ cup heavy cream
- 2 cups chicken stock
- Pepper
- Salt

Directions:

Add broccoli, stock, heavy cream, cream cheese, and butter to the slow cooker and stir well.
1. Cover and cook on high for 1 hour 30 minutes.
2. Stir well and add remaining ingredients and cook for 1 hour more.

3. Serve and enjoy.

Nutritional Value (Amount per Serving):

Calories 444

Fat 37 g

Carbohydrates 10 g

Sugar 2.5 g

Protein 20 g Cholesterol 116mg

Hearty Cabbage Beef Soup

Preparation Time: 10 minutes Cooking Time: 45 minutes

Serve: 10

Ingredients:

- 2 lbs ground beef
- 4 cups chicken stock
- 10 oz Rotel tomatoes, diced
- 3 cube bouillon
- 1 large cabbage head, chopped
- ½ tsp cumin powder
- 2 garlic cloves, minced
- ¼ onion, diced
- Pepper
- Salt

Directions:

1. Brown the meat in pan over medium heat.
2. Add onion and cook until soften.
3. Transfer meat mixture to the stock pot.
4. Add remaining ingredients to the stock pot stir well and bring to boil over high heat.
5. Turn heat to medium-low and simmer for 45 minutes.

Nutritional Value (Amount per Serving):

Calories 260

Fat 18 g

Carbohydrates 5 g

Sugar 2 g

Protein 15 g

Cholesterol 64 mg

Tasty Taco Soup

Preparation Time: 10 minutes Cooking Time: 4 hours

Serve: 8

Ingredients:

- 2 lbs ground beef
- 2 tbsp fresh cilantro, chopped
- 4 cups chicken stock
- 2 tbsp taco seasoning
- 20 oz Rotel
- 16 oz cream cheese

Directions:

1. Brown meat until fully cooked.
2. Transfer cooked meat in slow cooker.
3. Add remaining ingredients and stir well.
4. Cover and cook on low for 4 hours.
5. Stir well and serve.

Nutritional Value (Amount per Serving):

Calories 547

Fat 43 g

Carbohydrates 5 g

Sugar 4 g

Protein 33 g

Cholesterol 42 mg

BRUNCH & DINNER

Olive Cheese Omelet

Preparation Time: 10 minutes Cooking Time: 5 minutes
Serve: 4

Ingredients:

- 4 large eggs
- 2 oz cheese
- 12 olives, pitted
- 2 tbsp butter
- 2 tbsp olive oil
- 1 tsp herb de Provence
- 1/2 tsp salt

Directions:

1. Add all ingredients except butter in a bowl whisk well until frothy.
2. Melt butter in a pan over medium heat.
3. Pour egg mixture onto hot pan and spread evenly.
4. Cover and cook for 3 minutes.
5. Turn omelet to other side and cook for 2 minutes more.

6. Serve and enjoy.

Nutritional Value (Amount per Serving):

Calories 250

Fat 23 g

Carbohydrates 2 g

Sugar 1 g

Protein 10 g

Cholesterol 216 mg

Cheese Almond Pancakes

Preparation Time: 10 minutes Cooking Time: 10 minutes Serve: 4

Ingredients:

- 4 eggs
- 1/4 tsp cinnamon
- 1/2 cup cream cheese
- 1/2 cup almond flour
- 1 tbsp butter, melted

Directions:

1. Add all ingredients into the blender and blend until combined.
2. Melt butter in a pan over medium heat.
3. Pour 3 tablespoons of batter per pancake and cook for 2 minutes on each side.
4. Serve and enjoy.

Nutritional Value (Amount per Serving):

Calories 271

Fat 25 g

Carbohydrates 5 g

Sugar 1 g

Protein 10.8 g

Cholesterol 203 mg

DESSERTS & DRINKS

Cinnamon Almond Balls

Preparation Time: 10 minutes Cooking Time: 5 minutes Serve: 12

Ingredients:

- 1 tsp cinnamon
- 3 tbsp erythritol
- 1 ¼ cup almond flour
- 1 cup peanut butter
- Pinch of salt

Directions:

1. Add all ingredients into the mixing bowl and mix well.
2. Cover and place bowl in fridge for 30 minutes.
3. Make small bite size ball from mixture and serve.

Nutritional Value (Amount per Serving):

Calories 160

Fat 12 g

Carbohydrates 5 g

Sugar 1 g

Protein 6 g

Cholesterol 0 mg

Choco Frosty

Preparation Time: 5 minutes Cooking Time: 5 minutes

Serve: 4

Ingredients:

- 1 tsp vanilla
- 8 drops liquid stevia
- 2 tbsp unsweetened cocoa powder
- 1 tbsp almond butter
- 1 cup heavy cream

Directions:

1. Add all ingredients into the mixing bowl and beat with immersion blender until soft peaks form.
2. Place in refrigerator for 30 minutes.
3. Add frosty mixture into the piping bag and pipe in serving glasses.
4. Serve and enjoy.

Nutritional Value (Amount per Serving):

Calories 240

Fat 25 g

Carbohydrates 4 g

Sugar 3 g

Protein 3 g

Cholesterol 43 mg

Cheesecake Fat Bombs

Preparation Time: 10 minutes Cooking Time: 10 minutes

Serve: 24

Ingredients:

- 8 oz cream cheese
- 1 ½ tsp vanilla
- 2 tbsp erythritol
- 4 oz coconut oil
- 4 oz heavy cream

Directions:

1. Add all ingredients into the mixing bowl and beat using immersion blender until creamy.
2. Pour batter into the mini cupcake liner and place in refrigerator until set.
3. Serve and enjoy.

Nutritional Value (Amount per Serving):

Calories 90

Fat 9.8 g

Carbohydrates 1.4 g

Sugar 0.1 g

Protein 0.8 g

Cholesterol 17 mg

BREAKFAST RECIPES

Cheesy Ham Souffle

Serves: 4

Prep Time: 30 mins

Ingredients

- 1 cup cheddar cheese, shredded
- ½ cup heavy cream
- 6 large eggs
- 6 ounces ham, diced
- Salt and black pepper, to taste

Directions

1. Preheat the oven to 3500F and grease 4 ramekins gently.
2. Whisk together eggs in a medium bowl and add all other ingredients.
3. Mix well and pour the mixture into the ramekins.
4. Transfer into the ramekins and bake for about 18 minutes.
5. Remove from the oven and allow to slightly cool and serve.

Nutrition Amount per serving

Calories 342

Total Fat 26g 33% Saturated Fat 13g 65%

Cholesterol 353mg 118%

Sodium 841mg 37%

Total Carbohydrate 3g 1% Dietary Fiber 0.6g 2%

Total Sugars 0.8g

Protein 23.8g

Browned Butter Pumpkin Latte

Serves: 2

Prep Time: 10 mins

Ingredients

- 2 shots espresso
- 2 tablespoons butter
- 2 scoops Stevia
- 2 cups hot almond milk
- 4 tablespoons pumpkin puree

Directions

1. Heat butter on low heat in a small pan and allow to lightly brown.
2. Brew two shots of espresso and stir in the Stevia.
3. Add browned butter along with pumpkin puree and hot almond milk.
4. Blend for about 10 seconds on high and pour into 2 cups to serve.

Nutrition Amount per serving

Calories 227

Total Fat 22.6g 29% Saturated Fat 18.3g 92%

Cholesterol 31mg 10%

Sodium 93mg 4%

Total Carbohydrate 4.5g 2% Dietary Fiber 0.9g 3%

Total Sugars 1g, Protein 1.5g

Cauliflower Toast with Avocado

Serves: 2

Prep Time: 20 mins

Ingredients

- 1 large egg
- 1 small head cauliflower, grated
- 1 medium avocado, pitted and chopped
- ¾ cup mozzarella cheese, shredded
- Salt and black pepper, to taste

Directions

1. Preheat the oven to 420°F and line a baking sheet with parchment.
2. Place the cauliflower in a microwave safe bowl and microwave for about 7 minutes on high.
3. Spread on paper towels to drain after the cauliflower has completely cooled and press with a clean towel to remove excess moisture.
4. Put the cauliflower back in the bowl and stir in the mozzarella cheese and egg.
5. Season with salt and black pepper and stir until well combined.
6. Spoon the mixture onto the baking sheet in two rounded squares, as evenly as possible.
7. Bake for about 20 minutes until golden brown on the edges.

8. Mash the avocado with a pinch of salt and black pepper.
9. Spread the avocado onto the cauliflower toast and serve.

Nutrition Amount per serving

Calories 127 Total Fat 7g 9%

Saturated Fat 2.4g 12% Cholesterol 99mg 33%

Sodium 139mg 6%

Total Carbohydrate 9.1g 3% Dietary Fiber 4.8g 17% Total Sugars 3.4g

Protein 9.3g

Breakfast Cheesy Sausage

Serves: 1

Prep Time: 20 mins

Ingredients

- 1 pork sausage link, cut open and casing discarded
- Sea salt and black pepper, to taste
- ¼ teaspoon thyme
- ¼ teaspoon sage
- ½ cup mozzarella cheese, shredded

Directions

1. Mix sausage meat with thyme, sage, mozzarella cheese, sea salt and black pepper.
2. Shape the mixture into a patty and transfer to a hot pan.
3. Cook for about 5 minutes per side and dish out to serve.

Nutrition Amount per serving

Calories 91

Total Fat 7.1g 9% Saturated Fat 3g 15%

Cholesterol 17mg 6%

Sodium 218mg 9% Total Carbohydrate 1.1g

Dietary Fiber 0.2g 1% Total Sugars 0.2g

APPETIZERS AND DESSERTS

Caprese Snack

Serves: 4

Prep Time: 5 mins

Ingredients

- 8 oz. mozzarella, mini cheese balls
- 8 oz. cherry tomatoes
- 2 tablespoons green pesto
- Salt and black pepper, to taste
- 1 tablespoon garlic powder

Directions

1. Slice the mozzarella balls and tomatoes in half.
2. Stir in the green pesto and season with garlic powder, salt and pepper to serve.

Nutrition Amount per serving

Calories 407

Total Fat 34.5g 44% Saturated Fat 7.4g 37%

Cholesterol 30mg 10%

Sodium 343mg 15%

Total Carbohydrate 6.3g 2% Dietary Fiber 0.9g 3%

Total Sugars 2g Protein 19.4g

Almond Flour Crackers

Serves: 6

Prep Time: 25 mins

Ingredients

- 2 tablespoons sunflower seeds
- 1 cup almond flour
- ¾ teaspoon sea salt
- 1 tablespoon whole psyllium husks
- 1 tablespoon coconut oil

Directions

1. Preheat the oven to 3500F and grease a baking sheet lightly.
2. Mix together sunflower seeds, almond flour, sea salt, coconut oil, psyllium husks and 2 tablespoons of water in a bowl.
3. Transfer into a blender and blend until smooth.
4. Form a dough out of this mixture and roll it on the parchment paper until 1/16 inch thick.
5. Slice into 1 inch squares and season with some sea salt.
6. Arrange the squares on the baking sheet and transfer to the oven.
7. Bake for about 15 minutes until edges are crisp and brown.

8. Allow to cool and separate into squares to serve.

Nutrition Amount per serving

Calories 141

Total Fat 11.6g 15% Saturated Fat 2.7g 13%

Cholesterol 0mg 0%

Sodium 241mg 10%

Total Carbohydrate 5.2g 2% Dietary Fiber 3.1g

11% Total Sugars 0g

Protein 4.2g

PORK AND BEEF RECIPES

Hamburger Patties

Serves: 6

Prep Time: 30 mins

Ingredients

- 1 egg
- 25 oz. ground beef
- 3 oz. feta cheese, crumbled
- 2 oz. butter, for frying
- Salt and black pepper, to taste

Directions

1. Mix together egg, ground beef, feta cheese, salt and black pepper in a bowl.
2. Combine well and form equal sized patties.
3. Heat butter in a pan and add patties.
4. Cook on medium low heat for about 3 minutes per side.
5. Dish out and serve warm.

Nutrition Amount per serving

Calories 335

Total Fat 18.8g 24% Saturated Fat 10g 50%

Cholesterol 166mg 55%

Sodium 301mg 13%

Total Carbohydrate 0.7g 0% Dietary Fiber 0g 0%

Total Sugars 0.7g Protein 38.8g

Buttery Beef Curry

Serves: 2

Prep Time: 30 mins

Ingredients

- ½ cup butter
- ½ pound grass fed beef
- ½ pound onions
- Salt and red chili powder, to taste
- ½ pound celery, chopped

Directions

1. Put some water in a pressure cooker and add all the ingredients.
2. Lock the lid and cook on High Pressure for about 15 minutes.
3. Naturally release the pressure and dish out the curry to a bowl to serve.

Nutrition Amount per serving

Calories 450

Total Fat 38.4g 49% Saturated Fat 22.5g 113%

Cholesterol 132mg 44%

Sodium 340mg 15%

Total Carbohydrate 9.8g 4% Dietary Fiber 3.1g

11% Total Sugars 4.3g

Protein 17.2g

Cheesy Beef

Serves: 6

Prep Time: 40 mins

Ingredients

- 1 teaspoon garlic salt
- 2 pounds beef
- 1 cup cream cheese
- 1 cup mozzarella cheese, shredded
- 1 cup low carb Don Pablo's sauce

Directions

1. Season the meat with garlic salt and add to the instant pot.
2. Put the remaining ingredients in the pot and set the instant pot on low.
3. Cook for about 2 hours and dish out.

Nutrition Amount per serving

Calories 471

Total Fat 27.7g 36% Saturated Fat 14.6g 73%

Cholesterol 187mg 62%

Sodium 375mg 16%

Total Carbohydrate 2.9g 1% Dietary Fiber 0.1g 0%

Total Sugars 1.5g Protein 50.9g

Beef Quiche

Serves: 3

Prep Time: 30 mins

Ingredients

- ¼ cup grass fed beef, minced
- 2 slices bacon, cooked and crumbled
- ¼ cup goat cheddar cheese, shredded
- ¼ cup coconut milk
- 3 large pastured eggs

Directions

1. Preheat the oven to 3650F and grease 3 quiche molds.
2. Whisk together eggs and coconut milk in a large bowl.
3. Put beef in quiche molds and stir in the egg mixture.
4. Top with the crumbled bacon and cheddar cheese.
5. Transfer quiche molds to the oven and bake for about 20 minutes.
6. Remove from the oven and serve warm.

Nutrition Amount per serving

Calories 293

Total Fat 21.4g 27% Saturated Fat 10.4g 52% Cholesterol 232mg 77%

Sodium 436mg 19%

Total Carbohydrate 2.7g 1% Dietary Fiber 0.4g 2%

Total Sugars 1.1g Protein 21.8g

Chili Beef

Serves: 8

Prep Time: 50 mins

Ingredients

- 3 celery ribs, finely diced
- 2 pounds grass fed beef, ground
- 2 tablespoons chili powder
- 2 tablespoons avocado oil, divided
- 2 cups grass fed beef broth

Directions

1. Heat avocado oil in a skillet on medium heat and add beef.
2. Sauté for about 3 minutes on each side and stir in broth and chili powder.
3. Cover the lid and cook for about 30 minutes on medium low heat.
4. Add celery and dish out in a bowl to serve.

Nutrition Amount per serving

Calories 223

Total Fat 11.8g 15% Saturated Fat 4.7g 23%

Cholesterol 75mg 25%

Sodium 198mg 9%

Total Carbohydrate 2.4g 1% Dietary Fiber 1.2g 4%

Total Sugars 0.5g Protein 24.8g

SEAFOOD RECIPES

Garlic Butter Salmon

Serves: 8

Prep Time: 40 mins

Ingredients

- Kosher salt and black pepper, to taste
- 1 pound (3 pounds) salmon fillet, skin removed
- 4 tablespoons butter, melted
- 2 garlic cloves, minced
- ¼ cup parmesan cheese, freshly grated

Directions

1. Preheat the oven to 3500F and lightly grease a large baking sheet.
2. Season the salmon with salt and black pepper and transfer to the baking sheet.
3. Mix together butter, garlic and parmesan cheese in a small bowl.
4. Marinate salmon in this mixture for about 1 hour.
5. Transfer to the oven and bake for about 25 minutes.
6. Additionally, broil for about 2 minutes until top becomes lightly golden.
7. Dish out onto a platter and serve hot.

Nutrition Amount per serving

Calories 172

Total Fat 12.3g 16% Saturated Fat 6.2g 31%

Cholesterol 50mg 17%

Sodium 196mg 9%

Total Carbohydrate 0.8g 0% Dietary Fiber 0g 0%

Total Sugars 0g Protein 15.6g

Tuscan Butter Salmon

Serves: 4

Prep Time: 35 mins

Ingredients

- 4 (6 oz) salmon fillets, patted dry with paper towels
- 3 tablespoons butter
- ¾ cup heavy cream
- Kosher salt and black pepper
- 2 cups baby spinach

Directions

1. Season the salmon with salt and black pepper.
2. Heat 1½ tablespoons butter over medium high heat in a large skillet and add salmon skin side up.
3. Cook for about 10 minutes on both sides until deeply golden and dish out onto a plate.
4. Heat the rest of the butter in the skillet and add spinach.
5. Cook for about 5 minutes and stir in the heavy cream.
6. Reduce heat to low and simmer for about 3 minutes.
7. Return the salmon to the skillet and mix well with the sauce.
8. Allow to simmer for about 3 minutes until salmon is cooked through.
9. Dish out and serve hot.

Nutrition Amount per serving

Calories 382

Total Fat 27.5g 35% Saturated Fat 12.2g 61%

Cholesterol 129mg 43%

Sodium 157mg 7%

Total Carbohydrate 1.2g 0% Dietary Fiber 0.3g 1%

Total Sugars 0.1g Protein 34g

Mahi Mahi Stew

Serves: 3

Prep Time: 45 mins

Ingredients

- 2 tablespoons butter
- 2 pounds Mahi Mahi fillets, cubed
- 1 onion, chopped
- Salt and black pepper, to taste
- 2 cups homemade fish broth

Directions

1. Season the Mahi Mahi fillets with salt and black pepper.
2. Heat butter in a pressure cooker and add onion.
3. Sauté for about 3 minutes and stir in the seasoned Mahi Mahi fillets and fish broth.
4. Lock the lid and cook on High Pressure for about 30 minutes.
5. Naturally release the pressure and dish out to serve hot.

Nutrition Amount per serving

Calories 398

Total Fat 12.5g 16% Saturated Fat 6.4g 32% Cholesterol 290mg 97%

Sodium 803mg 35%

Total Carbohydrate 5.5g 2% Dietary Fiber 1.5g 5%

Total Sugars 2.2g Protein 62.3g

VEGAN & VEGETARIAN

Browned Butter Cauliflower Mash

Serves: 4

Prep Time: 35 mins

Ingredients

- 1 yellow onion, finely chopped
- ¾ cup heavy whipping cream
- 1½ pounds cauliflower, shredded
- Sea salt and black pepper, to taste
- 3½ oz. butter

Directions

1. Heat 2 tablespoons butter in a skillet on medium heat and add onions.
2. Sauté for about 3 minutes and dish out to a bowl.
3. Mix together cauliflower, heavy whipping cream, sea salt and black pepper in the same skillet.
4. Cover with lid and cook on medium low heat for about 15 minutes.
5. Season with salt and black pepper and stir in sautéed onions.
6. Dish out to a bowl and heat the rest of the butter in the skillet.
7. Cook until the butter is brown and nutty and serve with cauliflower mash.

Nutrition Amount per serving

Calories 309

Total Fat 28.7g 37% Saturated Fat 18g 90%

Cholesterol 84mg 28%

Sodium 204mg 9%

Total Carbohydrate 12.2g 4% Dietary Fiber 4.8g 17%

Total Sugars 5.3g Protein 4.3g

Cauliflower Gratin

Serves: 6

Prep Time: 35 mins

Ingredients

- 20 oz. cauliflower, chopped
- 2 oz. salted butter, for frying
- 5 oz. cheddar cheese, shredded
- 15 oz. sausages in links, precooked and chopped into 1 inch pieces
- 1 cup crème fraiche

Directions

1. Preheat the oven to 3750F and grease a baking dish lightly.
2. Heat 1 oz. butter in a pan on medium low heat and add chopped cauliflower.
3. Sauté for about 4 minutes and transfer to the baking dish.
4. Heat the rest of the butter in a pan on medium low heat and add sausage links.
5. Sauté for about 3 minutes and transfer to the baking dish on top of cauliflower.
6. Pour the crème fraiche in the baking dish and top with cheddar cheese.
7. Transfer into the oven and bake for about 15 minutes.

8. Dish out to a bowl and serve hot.

Nutrition Amount per serving

Calories 509

Total Fat 43.7g 56% Saturated Fat 21.3g 107%

Cholesterol 122mg 41%

Sodium 781mg 34%

Total Carbohydrate 7g 3% Dietary Fiber 2.4g 8%

Total Sugars 2.5g

Protein 22.8g

CHICKEN AND POULTRY RECIPES

Turkey with Cream Cheese Sauce

Serves: 4

Prep Time: 30 mins

Ingredients

- 20 oz. turkey breast
- 2 tablespoons butter
- 2 cups heavy whipping cream
- Salt and black pepper, to taste
- 7 oz. cream cheese

Directions

1. Season the turkey generously with salt and black pepper.
2. Heat butter in a skillet over medium heat and cook turkey for about 5 minutes on each side.
3. Stir in the heavy whipping cream and cream cheese.
4. Cover the skillet and cook for about 15 minutes on medium low heat.
5. Dish out to serve hot.

Nutrition Amount per serving

Calories 386
Total Fat 31.7g 41% Saturated Fat 19.2g 96%
Cholesterol 142mg 47%
Sodium 1100mg 48% Total Carbohydrate 6g 2%
Dietary Fiber 0.5g 2% Total Sugars 3.4g
Protein 19.5g

Keto Pesto Chicken Casserole

Serves: 3

Prep Time: 45 mins

Ingredients

- 1½ pounds boneless chicken thighs, cut into bite sized pieces
- Salt and black pepper, to taste
- 2 tablespoons butter
- 3 oz. green pesto
- 5 oz. feta cheese, diced

Directions

1. Preheat the oven to 400 F and grease a baking dish.
2. Season the chicken with salt and black pepper.
3. Heat butter in a skillet over medium heat and cook chicken for about 5 minutes on each side.
4. Dish out in the greased baking dish and add feta cheese and pesto.
5. Transfer the baking dish to the oven and bake for about 30 minutes.
6. Remove from the oven and serve hot.

Nutrition Amount per serving

Calories 438

Total Fat 30.4g 39% Saturated Fat 11g 55%

Cholesterol 190mg 63%

Sodium 587mg 26%

Total Carbohydrate 1.7g 1% Dietary Fiber 0g 0%

Total Sugars 1.5g Protein 39.3g

BREAKFAST RECIPES

Cauliflower Zucchini Fritters

Total Time: 15 minutes Serves: 4

Ingredients:

- 3 cups cauliflower florets
- ¼ tsp black pepper
- ¼ cup coconut flour
- 2 medium zucchini, grated and squeezed
- 1 tbsp coconut oil
- ½ tsp sea salt

Directions:

1. Steam cauliflower florets for 5 minutes.
2. Add cauliflower into the food processor and process until it looks like rice.
3. Add all ingredients except coconut oil to the large bowl and mix until well combined.
4. Make small round patties from the mixture and set aside.
5. Heat coconut oil in a pan over medium heat.
6. Place patties on pan and cook for 3-4 minutes on each side.

7. Serve and enjoy.

Nutritional Value (Amount per Serving): Calories 68; Fat 3.8 g; Carbohydrates 7.8 g;

Sugar 3.6 g; Protein 2.8 g; Cholesterol 0 mg;

Flax Almond Muffins

Total Time: 45 minutes Serves: 6

Ingredients:

- 1 tsp cinnamon
- 2 tbsp coconut flour
- 20 drops liquid stevia
- 1/4 cup water
- 1/4 tsp vanilla extract
- 1/4 tsp baking soda
- 1/2 tsp baking powder
- 1/4 cup almond flour
- 1/2 cup ground flax
- 2 tbsp ground chia

Directions:

Preheat the oven to 350 F/ 176 C.

1. Spray muffin tray with cooking spray and set aside.
2. In a small bowl, add 6 tablespoons of water and ground chia. Mix well and set aside.
3. In a mixing bowl, add ground flax, baking soda, baking powder, cinnamon, coconut flour, and almond flour and mix well.
4. Add chia seed mixture, vanilla, water, and liquid stevia and stir well to combine.
5. Pour mixture into the prepared muffin tray and bake in preheated oven for 35 minutes.
6. Serve and enjoy.

Nutritional Value (Amount per Serving): Calories 92; Fat 6.3 g; Carbohydrates 6.9 g; Sugar 0.4 g; Protein 3.7 g; Cholesterol 0 mg;

Fresh Berries with Cream

Total Time: 10 minutes Serves: 1

Ingredients:

- 1/2 cup coconut cream
- 1 oz strawberries
- 1 oz raspberries
- 1/4 tsp vanilla extract

Directions:

1. Add all ingredients into the blender and blend until smooth.
2. Pour in serving bowl and top with fresh berries.
3. Serve and enjoy.

Nutritional Value (Amount per Serving): Calories 303; Fat 28.9 g; Carbohydrates 12 g; Sugar 6.8 g; Protein 3.3 g; Cholesterol 0 mg;

Chia Flaxseed Waffles

Total Time: 25 minutes Serves: 8

Ingredients:

- 2 cups ground golden flaxseed
- 2 tsp cinnamon
- 10 tsp ground chia seed
- 15 tbsp warm water
- 1/3 cup coconut oil, melted
- 1/2 cup water
- 1 tbsp baking powder
- 1 tsp sea salt

Directions:

1. Preheat the waffle iron.
2. In a small bowl, mix together ground chia seed and warm water.
3. In a large bowl, mix together ground flax seed, sea salt, and baking powder. Set aside.
4. Add melted coconut oil, chia seed mixture, and water into the blender and blend for 30 seconds.
5. Transfer coconut oil mixture into the flax seed mixture and mix well. Add cinnamon and stir well.
6. Scoop waffle mixture into the hot waffle iron and cook on each side for 3-5 minutes.
7. Serve and enjoy.

Nutritional Value (Amount per Serving):

Calories 240; Fat 20.6 g; Carbohydrates 12.9 g; Sugar 0 g; Protein 7 g; Cholesterol 0 mg;

Cinnamon Noatmeal

Total Time: 10 minutes Serves: 2

Ingredients:

- ¾ cup hot water
- 2 tbsp sugar-free maple syrup
- ½ tsp ground cinnamon
- 2 tbsp ground flax seeds
- 3 tbsp vegan vanilla protein powder
- 3 tbsp hulled hemp seeds

Directions:

1. Add all ingredients into the bowl and stir until well combined.
2. Serve and enjoy.

Nutritional Value (Amount per Serving): Calories 220; Fat 12.5 g; Carbohydrates 9.5 g; Sugar 0.1 g; Protein 17.6 g; Cholesterol 0 mg;

LUNCH RECIPES

Herb Spaghetti Squash

Total Time: minutes Serves: 4

Ingredients:

- 4 cups spaghetti squash, cooked
- ½ tsp pepper
- ½ tsp sage
- 1 tsp dried parsley
- 1 tsp dried thyme
- 1 tsp dried rosemary
- 1 tsp garlic powder
- 2 tbsp olive oil
- 1 tsp salt

Directions:

1. Preheat the oven to 350 F/ 180 C.
2. Add all ingredients into the mixing bowl and mix well to combine.
3. Transfer bowl mixture to the oven safe dish and cook in preheated oven for 15 minutes.
4. Stir well and serve.

Nutritional Value (Amount per Serving): Calories 96; Fat 7.7 g; Carbohydrates 8.1 g;

Sugar 0.2 g; Protein 0.9 g; Cholesterol 0 mg;

Delicious Cabbage Steaks

Total Time: 1 hour 10 minutes

Serves: 6

Ingredients:

- 1 medium cabbage head, slice 1" thick
- 2 tbsp olive oil
- 1 tbsp garlic, minced
- Pepper
- Salt

Directions:

1. In a small bowl, mix together garlic and olive oil.
2. Brush garlic and olive oil mixture onto both sides of sliced cabbage.
3. Season cabbage slices with pepper and salt.
4. Place cabbage slices onto a baking tray and bake at 350 F/ 180 C for 1 hour. Turn after 30 minutes.
5. Serve and enjoy.

Nutritional Value (Amount per Serving): Calories 72; Fat 4.8 g; Carbohydrates 7.4 g;
Sugar 3.8 g; Protein 1.6 g; Cholesterol 0 mg;

Mexican Cauliflower Rice

Total Time: 25 minutes Serves: 4

Ingredients:

- 1 medium cauliflower head, cut into florets
- ½ cup tomato sauce
- ¼ tsp black pepper
- 1 tsp chili powder
- 2 garlic cloves, minced
- ½ medium onion, diced
- 1 tbsp coconut oil
- ½ tsp sea sal

Directions:

1. Add cauliflower florets into the food processor and process until it looks like rice.
2. Heat oil in a pan over medium-high heat.
3. Add onion to the pan and sauté for 5 minutes or until softened.
4. Add garlic and cook for 1 minute.
5. Add cauliflower rice, chili powder, pepper, and salt. Stir well.
6. Add tomato sauce and cook for 5 minutes.
7. Stir well and serve warm.

Nutritional Value (Amount per Serving): Calories 83; Fat 3.7g; Carbohydrates 11.5 g; Sugar 5.4 g; Protein 3.6 g; Cholesterol 0 mg;

Asparagus Mash

Total Time: 20 minutes Serves: 2

Ingredients:

- 10 asparagus shoots, chopped
- 1 tsp lemon juice
- 2 tbsp fresh parsley
- 2 tbsp coconut cream
- 1 small onion, diced
- 1 tbsp coconut oil
- Pepper
- Salt

Directions:

1. Sauté onion in coconut oil until onion is softened.
2. Blanch chopped asparagus in hot water for 2 minutes and drain immediately.
3. Add sautéed onion, lemon juice, parsley, coconut cream, asparagus, pepper, and salt into the blender and blend until smooth.
4. Serve warm and enjoy.

Nutritional Value (Amount per Serving): Calories 125; Fat 10.6 g; Carbohydrates 7.5 g; Sugar 3.6 g; Protein 2.6 g; Cholesterol 0 mg;

Creamy Squash Soup

Total Time: 35 minutes Serves: 8

Ingredients:

- 3 cups butternut squash, chopped
- 1 ½ cups unsweetened coconut milk
- 1 tbsp coconut oil
- 1 tsp dried onion flakes
- 1 tbsp curry powder
- 4 cups water
- 1 garlic clove
- 1 tsp kosher salt

Directions:

1. Add squash, coconut oil, onion flakes, curry powder, water, garlic, and salt into a large saucepan. Bring to boil over high heat.
2. Turn heat to medium and simmer for 20 minutes.
3. Puree the soup using a blender until smooth. Return soup to the saucepan and stir in coconut milk and cook for 2 minutes.
4. Stir well and serve hot.

Nutritional Value (Amount per Serving): Calories 146; Fat 12.6 g; Carbohydrates 9.4 g; Sugar 2.8 g; Protein 1.7 g; Cholesterol 0 mg;

Spinach with Coconut Milk

Total Time: 25 minutes Serves: 6

Ingredients:

- 16 oz spinach
- 2 tsp curry powder
- 13.5 oz coconut milk
- 1 tsp lemon zest
- ½ tsp salt

Directions:

1. Add spinach in pan and heat over medium heat. Once it is hot then add curry paste and few tablespoons of coconut milk. Stir well.
2. Add remaining coconut milk, lemon zest, and salt and cook until thickened.
3. Serve and enjoy.

Nutritional Value (Amount per Serving): Calories 167; Fat 15.6 g; Carbohydrates 6.7 g; Sugar 2.5 g; Protein 3.7 g; Cholesterol 0 mg;

DINNER RECIPES

Roasted Squash

Total Time: 1 hour 10 minutes

Serves: 3

Ingredients:

- 2 lbs. summer squash, cut into 1-inch pieces
- 1/8 tsp pepper
- 1/8 tsp garlic powder
- 3 tbsp olive oil
- 1 large lemon juice
- 1/8 tsp paprika
- Pepper
- Salt

Directions:

1. Preheat the oven to 400 F/ 204 C.
2. Spray a baking tray with cooking spray.
3. Place squash pieces onto the prepared baking tray and drizzle with olive oil.
4. Season with paprika, pepper, and garlic powder.
5. Squeeze lemon juice over the squash and bake in preheated oven for 50-60 minutes.
6. Serve hot and enjoy.

Nutritional Value (Amount per Serving): Calories 182; Fat 15 g; Carbohydrates 12.3 g; Sugar 11 g; Protein 3.2 g; Cholesterol 0 mg;

Lemon Garlic Mushrooms

Total Time: 25 minutes Serves: 4

Ingredients:

- 3 oz enoki mushrooms
- 1 tbsp olive oil
- 1 tsp lemon zest, chopped
- 2 tbsp lemon juice
- 3 garlic cloves, sliced
- 6 oyster mushrooms, halved
- 5 oz cremini mushrooms, sliced
- 1/2 red chili, sliced
- 1/2 onion, sliced
- 1 tsp sea salt

Directions:

1. Heat olive oil in a pan over high heat.
2. Add shallots, enoki mushrooms, oyster mushrooms, cremini mushrooms, and chili.
3. Stir well and cook over medium-high heat for 10 minutes.
4. Add lemon zest and stir well. Season with lemon juice and salt and cook for 3-4 minutes.
5. Serve and enjoy.

Nutritional Value (Amount per Serving): Calories 87; Fat 5.6 g; Carbohydrates 7.5 g;

Sugar 1.8 g; Protein 3 g; Cholesterol 8 mg;

Almond Green Beans

Total Time: 20 minutes Serves: 4

Ingredients:

- 1 lb fresh green beans, trimmed
- 1/3 cup almonds, sliced
- 4 garlic cloves, sliced
- 2 tbsp olive oil
- 1 tbsp lemon juice
- ½ tsp sea salt

Directions:

1. Add green beans, salt, and lemon juice in a mixing bowl. Toss well and set aside.
2. Heat oil in a pan over medium heat.
3. Add sliced almonds and sauté until lightly browned.
4. Add garlic and sauté for 30 seconds.
5. Pour almond mixture over green beans and toss well.
6. Stir well and serve immediately.

Nutritional Value (Amount per Serving): Calories 146; Fat 11.2 g; Carbohydrates 10.9 g; Sugar 2 g; Protein 4 g; Cholesterol 0 mg;

Fried Okra

Total Time: 20 minutes Serves: 4

Ingredients:

- 1 lb fresh okra, cut into ¼" slices
- 1/3 cup almond meal
- Pepper
- Salt
- Oil for frying

Directions:

1. Heat oil in large pan over medium- high heat.
2. In a bowl, mix together sliced okra, almond meal, pepper, and salt until well coated.
3. Once the oil is hot then add okra to the hot oil and cook until lightly browned.
4. Remove fried okra from pan and allow to drain on paper towels.
5. Serve and enjoy.

Nutritional Value (Amount per Serving): Calories 91; Fat 4.2 g; Carbohydrates 10.2 g; Sugar 10.2 g; Protein 3.9 g; Cholesterol 0 mg;

DESSERT RECIPES

Lemon Mousse

Total Time: 10 minutes Serves: 2

Ingredients:

- 14 oz coconut milk
- 12 drops liquid stevia
- 1/2 tsp lemon extract
- 1/4 tsp turmeric

Directions:

1. Place coconut milk can in the refrigerator for overnight. Scoop out thick cream into a mixing bowl.
2. Add remaining ingredients to the bowl and whip using a hand mixer until smooth.
3. Transfer mousse mixture to a zip-lock bag and pipe into small serving glasses. Place in refrigerator.
4. Serve chilled and enjoy.

Nutritional Value (Amount per Serving): Calories 444; Fat 45.7 g; Carbohydrates 10 g; Sugar 6 g; Protein 4.4 g; Cholesterol 0 mg;

BREAKFAST RECIPES

Almond Butter Shake

Get your morning started right with this fantastic boost in energy that takes just 5 minutes to make.

Total Prep & Cooking Time: 5 minutes Level: Beginner

Makes: 1 Shake

Protein: 19 grams Net Carbs: 6 grams Fat: 27 grams

Sugar: 0 grams

Calories: 326

What you need:

- 1 1/2 cups almond milk, unsweetened
- 2 tbs almond butter
- 1/2 tbs ground cinnamon
- 2 tbs flax meal
- 1/8 tsp almond extract, sugar-free
- 15 drops liquid Stevia
- 1/8 tsp salt
- 6 ice cubes

Steps:

Using a blender, combine all the listed ingredients and pulse for approximately 45 seconds.

Serve immediately and enjoy!

Bacon & Egg Fat Bomb

Healthy packed breakfast fat bombs that are guaranteed to satisfy you throughout the morning.

Total Prep & Cooking Time: 50 minutes Level: Beginner

Makes: 3 Fat Bombs Protein: 2 grams

Net Carbs: 0.1 grams Fat: 13 grams

Sugar: 0 grams

Calories: 127

What you need:

- 1 large egg
- 12 cups of cold water, separated
- 1/4 tsp salt
- 3 tsp mayonnaise, sugar-free
- 1/8 cup butter
- 2 slices bacon
- 1/8 tsp pepper

Steps:

1. Fill a pot with 6 cups of the cold water and the eggs.
2. Set the timer for 7 minutes once the water starts to boil.
3. When the time has passed, drain the water and pour the remaining 6 cups of cold water on the eggs to halt the heating process.
4. Once cooled, peel the eggs and place in a dish with the butter, pepper, mayonnaise, and salt, whisking until combined.
5. Refrigerate for approximately half an hour.
6. Heat the bacon in a skillet until crispy and brown. Place on a plate with paper towels.
7. Crumble the bacon once cooled onto a small plate and remove the eggs from the fridge.
8. Scoop out small balls and cover entirely in the bacon bits, and serve immediately.

LUNCH RECIPES

Avocado Chicken Salad

Enjoy this colorful mix of the customary chicken salad that is low in carbs and high in

potassium. Your heart will be thanking you.

Total Prep & Cooking Time: 15 minutes Level: Beginner

Makes: 4 Helpings

Protein: 14 grams Net Carbs: 0.4 grams Fat: 2 grams

Sugar: 0 grams

Calories: 74

What you need:

- 12.5 oz. canned chicken, drained and shredded
- 1 large avocado
- 8 oz. cilantro, chopped
- 1/4 tsp salt
- 8 oz. celery, chopped
- 1/8 tsp pepper

Steps:

1. Mash the avocado using a food blender for approximately half a minute. Combine the chicken, salt, chopped cilantro, chopped celery, and pepper and pulse until incorporated.
2. Transfer to a serving plate and enjoy.

Variation Tip:

Instead of canned chicken, you can use the same amount of rotisserie chicken. You can eat as is, place on a leaf of lettuce or a slice of low carb bread.

Burger Cabbage Stir Fry

This quick lunch dish is easy to whip up even in the morning so it can be brought with you to work.

Total Prep & Cooking Time: 20 minutes

Level: Beginner Makes: 4 Helpings

Protein: 9 grams

Net Carbs: 1.5 grams Fat: 8 grams

Sugar: 1 gram

Calories: 208

What you need:

- 1/4 tsp salt
- 5 oz. ground beef
- 1 tsp onion powder
- 8 oz. cabbage, sliced
- 1 clove garlic, minced
- 2 tbs coconut oil
- 1/8 tsp pepper

Steps:

1. In a big skillet, combine the bacon and beef and brown for approximately 7 minutes.
2. Then fry the minced garlic, chopped cabbage and onion powder with the meat for about 2 additional minutes.
3. Serve warm after seasoning with pepper and salt.

Baking Tip:

For this stir fry, you can also use a wok instead of the skillet.

SNACK

Bacon Wrapped Avocado

This quick fried snack is going to have you filling up on the nutrients and fats that your body craves.

Total Prep & Cooking Time: 30 minutes Level: Beginner

Makes: 3 Helpings (2 wraps per serving) Protein: 15 grams

Net Carbs: 1.8 grams Fat: 21 grams

Sugar: 0 grams

Calories: 139

What you need:

- 1 avocado, peeled and pitted
- 6 strips bacon
- 1 tbs butter

Steps:

1. Slice the avocado into 6 individual wedges.
2. Wrap one slice of bacon around the avocado wedge and repeat for all pieces.
3. Soften the butter in a non-stick skillet and transfer the wedges to the hot butter with the end of the bacon on the base of the pan. This will prevent the bacon from coming apart from the wedge.
4. Cook for approximately 3 minutes on each side, and move to a paper towel covered plate.
5. Serve while still hot and enjoy!

Baking Tip:

Do not use an avocado that is mushy or overripe as it will crumble while wrapping with the bacon.

Variation Tip:

You can also substitute asparagus instead of the avocado.

DINNER RECIPES

Beef & Broccoli Stir fry

This stir fry meal is very easy to throw together even on a weeknight and tastes oh so yummy.

Total Prep & Cooking Time: 20 minutes plus 1 hour to marinate

Level: Beginner

Makes: 4 Helpings

Protein: 24 grams Net Carbs: 6 grams Fat: 26 grams

Sugar: 1 gram

Calories: 192

What you need:

For the main dish:

- 1/4 cup coconut oil
- 16 oz. flat iron steak
- 1 tsp toasted sesame oil
- 8 oz. broccoli, florets
- 1 tsp fish sauce

For the marinade:

- 1/8 cup tamari sauce, gluten-free
- 2 cloves garlic, chopped
- 1 tsp ginger, grated

Steps:

1. Slice the steak into quarter-inch pieces by cutting against the grain.
2. In a ziplock bag, combine the beef, tamari sauce, chopped garlic, and grated ginger. Refrigerate for an hour to marinate.
3. Boil the broccoli in a saucepan for approximately 2 minutes and drain as much water as possible.
4. Meanwhile, in a large skillet or wok, melt the coconut oil.
5. Remove the beef from the marinade and reserve the sauce for later.
6. When the pan is very hot, brown the beef for approximately 2 minutes and remove the meat to a plate.
7. Fry the broccoli in the wok for about 3 minutes and empty the marinade liquid into the pan. Allow to heat for 2 additional minutes.
8. Transfer the beef to the wok for approximately 90 seconds, stirring occasionally.
9. Drizzle the toasted sesame oil and fish sauce over the contents of the pan and serve.

Baking Tip:

1. You may want to go straight to cooking without marinating the meat, but this will take away the amazing flavor that hour can give.

Variation Tips:

Alternatively, you can use sirloin or flank steak in place of the flat iron steak.

Beef Kheema Meatloaf

This is an excellent twist on the conventional meatloaf recipe that is a brilliant way to use up that ground beef in your freezer.

Total Prep & Cooking Time: 25 minutes Level: Beginner

Makes: 4 Helpings

Protein: 26 grams Net Carbs: 5 grams

Fat: 13 grams

Sugar: 1 gram

Calories: 260

What you need:

- 16 oz. ground beef
- 1 tsp turmeric
- 2 large eggs
- 1 tbs onion powder
- 4 oz. cilantro, chopped
- 1 tsp salt
- 3 tsp ginger, minced
- 1 tsp cayenne pepper
- 3 tsp garlic, minced
- 1/2 tsp ground cinnamon
- 2 tsp garam masala
- 1/8 tsp ground cardamom
- Air Fryer

Steps:

2. Set the temperature of the air fryer to heat at 360° Fahrenheit. Place an 8- inch heat safe round pan to the side.
3. In a food blender, combine all the listed components and pulse until thoroughly combined.
4. Distribute the meat evenly into the round pan and set the air fryer timer for 15 minutes.
5. After the time has passed, check with a meat thermometer to make sure it is at a uniform 160° Fahrenheit. If not, set for an additional 5 minutes.
6. Take out the pan and drain the meat.
7. Divide the meat into 4 equal servings and enjoy!

Baking Tip:

1. If garam masala is not available, you can make your own! Simply add 1/2 tablespoon allspice and 1 1/2 tablespoon cumin seasonings.

UNUSUAL DDELICIOUS MEAL RECIPES

You have made it to the bonus chapter where there is a unique collection of recipes, as most are exotic and from overseas. Some have a few more steps, but they are still going to be easy enough for anyone to bring to their dinner table tonight. Enjoy experimenting with something new!

Blackberry Clafoutis Tarts

This rendition of the traditional dessert from France is very creamy and low carb

to boot.

Total Prep & Cooking Time: 1 hour 30 minutes

Level: Beginner Makes: 4 Tarts

Protein: 3 grams

Net Carbs: 2.4 grams Fat: 15 grams

Sugar: 1 gram

Calories: 201

What you need:

For the crust:

- 1/4 cup coconut flour
- 2 tbs coconut oil, melted
- 2 tbs almond butter, smooth
- 1/4 tsp Swerve sweetener, confectioner
- 2 1/2 cups pecan pieces, raw
- 1/8 tsp salt

For the filling:

- 1 large egg
- 8 oz. blackberries
- 1/8 cup almond flour, blanched
- 2 oz. almond milk, unsweetened
- 3 tsp Stevia sweetener, granulated
- 1/8 tsp salt
- 3 oz. coconut milk, canned
- 1 tsp vanilla extract, sugar-free

Steps:

1. Set the stove to heat at 350° Fahrenheit. You will need to set aside four 4 3/4-inch tart pans.
2. To create the tart crusts, blend the coconut flour, Swerve, pecan pieces, salt, coconut oil, almond butter in a food blender for approximately 2 minutes until crumbly.
3. Scrape down the bowl with a rubber scraper and pulse

for an additional 30 seconds.
4. Portion the batter in 4 equal sections and distribute to the tart pans. Press the crust evenly by starting with the sides with the middle being pressed last. Refrigerate to set for half an hour.
5. Remove the crusts from the fridge and place a quarter cup of blackberries in each tart pan.
6. Using the food blender, whip the Stevia, vanilla extract, egg, salt, coconut milk and almond milk for approximately half a minute.
7. Empty the contents evenly over the blackberries.
8. Heat the tarts for about half an hour and remove to the counter.
9. Wait approximately 10 minutes for serving warm. Enjoy!

Calamari Salad

This meal might look a little bit too unusual, but it will build your muscles after that powerful workout.

Total Prep & Cooking Time: 10 minutes Level: Beginner

Makes: 4 Helpings

Protein: 18 grams Net Carbs: 5 grams

Fat: 14 grams

Sugar: 0 grams

Calories: 214

What you need:

- 1/2 tsp lime juice
- 16 oz. calamari, sliced
- 1/4 tsp salt
- 2 tbs coconut oil
- 1/8 tsp pepper
- 8 oz. olives
- 1/2 tsp garlic powder
- 3 tsp coconut oil, separate
- 1/2 tsp lemon juice

Steps:

1. In a glass dish, blend the lemon and lime juice fully.
2. In a separate dish, whisk the 3 teaspoons of coconut oil, salt, garlic powder, and pepper until combined.
3. In a non-stick skillet, dissolve the 2 tablespoons of coconut oil with the olives. Heat the olives for about 90 seconds and remove to a serving plate.
4. Coat the calamari liberally in the seasonings.
5. Transfer the calamari to the hot oil and stir fry for approximately 2 minutes or until they become cloudy.
6. Remove to the serving plate with the olives.
7. Drizzle the juice dressing over the top of the plate and serve.

KETO DESSERTS RECIPES

Pumpkin Bars

Serves: 16

Preparation time: 10 minutes Cooking time: 28 minutes

Ingredients:

- 2 eggs
- 1 ½ tsp pumpkin pie spice
- ½ tsp baking soda
- 1 tsp baking powder
- ¼ cup coconut flour
- 8 oz pumpkin puree
- ½ cup coconut oil, melted
- 1/3 cup Swerve
- Pinch of salt

Directions:

1. Preheat the oven to 350 F/ 180 C.
2. Spray 9*9 inch baking pan with cooking spray and set aside.
3. In a bowl, beat eggs, sweetener, coconut oil, pumpkin pie spice, and pumpkin puree until well combined.

4. In another bowl, mix together coconut flour, baking soda, baking powder, and salt.
5. Add coconut flour mixture to the egg mixture and mix well.
6. Pour bar mixture into the prepared baking pan and spread evenly.
7. Bake in preheated oven for 28 minutes.
8. Allow to cool completely then slice and serve.

Per Serving: Net Carbs: 1.1g; Calories: 73; Total Fat: 7.5g; Saturated Fat: 6.1g

Protein: 0.9g; Carbs: 1.6g; Fiber: 0.5g; Sugar: 0.5g; Fat 90% / Protein 4% / Carbs 6%

Flavors Pumpkin Bars

Serves: 18

Preparation time: 10 minutes Cooking time: 10 minutes

Ingredients:

- 1 tbsp coconut flour
- ½ tsp cinnamon
- 2 tsp pumpkin pie spice
- 1 tsp liquid stevia
- ½ cup erythritol
- 15 oz can pumpkin puree
- 15 oz can unsweetened coconut milk
- 16 oz cocoa butter

Directions:

1. Line baking dish with parchment paper and set aside.
2. Melt cocoa butter in a small saucepan over low heat.
3. Add pumpkin puree and coconut milk and stir well.
4. Add remaining ingredients and whisk well.
5. Stir the mixture continuously until mixture thickens.
6. Once the mixture thickens then pour it into prepared baking dish and place in the refrigerator for 2 hours.
7. Slice and serve.

Per Serving: Net Carbs: 5.8g; Calories: 282; Total Fat: 28.1g; Saturated Fat: 17.1g

Protein: 1.3g; Carbs: 9.5g; Fiber: 3.7g; Sugar: 4g; Fat 89% / Protein 2% / Carbs 9%

Coconut Lemon Bars

Serves: 24

Preparation time: 10 minutes Cooking time: 42 minutes

Ingredients:

- 4 eggs
- 1 tbsp coconut flour
- 3/4 cup Swerve
- 1/2 tsp baking powder
- 1/3 cup fresh lemon juice
- For crust:
- 1/4 cup Swerve
- 2 1/4 cups almond flour
- 1/2 cup coconut oil, melted

Directions:

1. Preheat the oven to 350 F/ 180 C.
2. Spray a baking dish with cooking spray and set aside.
3. In a small bowl, mix together 1/4 cup swerve and almond flour.
4. Add melted coconut oil and mix until it forms into a dough.
5. Transfer dough into the prepared pan and spread evenly.
6. Bake for 15 minutes.
7. For the filling: Add eggs, coconut flour, baking powder, lemon juice, and swerve into the blender and blend for 10 seconds.

8. Pour blended mixture on top of baked crust and spread well.
9. Bake for 25 minutes.
10. Remove from oven and set aside to cool completely.
11. Slice and serve.

Per Serving: Net Carbs: 1.5g; Calories: 113; Total Fat: 10.6g; Saturated Fat: 4.6g

Protein: 3.3g; Carbs: 2.8g; Fiber: 1.3g; Sugar: 0.5g; Fat 84% / Protein 11% / Carbs 5%

CAKE

Beginner:Delicious Ricotta Cake

Serves: 8

Preparation time: 10 minutes Cooking time: 45 minutes

Ingredients:

- 2 eggs
- ½ cup erythritol
- ¼ cup coconut flour
- 15 oz ricotta
- Pinch of salt

Directions:

1. Preheat the oven to 350 F/ 180 C.
2. Spray 9-inch baking pan with cooking spray and set aside.
3. In a bowl whisk eggs.
4. Add remaining ingredients and mix until well combined.
5. Transfer batter in prepared baking pan.
6. Bake in preheated oven for 45 minutes.
7. Remove baking pan from oven and allow to cool completely.
8. Slice and serve.

Per Serving: Net Carbs: 2.9g; Calories: 91; Total Fat: 5.4g; Saturated Fat: 3g

Protein: 7.5g; Carbs: 3.1g; Fiber: 0.2g; Sugar: 0.3g; Fat 55% / Protein 33% / Carbs 12%

Chocó Coconut Cake

Serves: 9

Preparation time: 10 minutes Cooking time: 25 minutes

Ingredients:

- 6 eggs
- 1 tsp vanilla
- 3 oz butter, melted
- oz heavy whipping cream
- 2 tsp baking powder
- 3 oz unsweetened cocoa powder
- 5 oz erythritol
- oz coconut flour

Directions:

1. Preheat the oven to 350 F/ 180 C.
2. In a bowl, mix together coconut flour, butter, 5.5 oz heavy whipping cream, eggs, baking powder 1.5 oz cocoa powder, and 3 oz erythritol until well combined.
3. Pour batter into the greased cake pan and bake in preheated oven for 25 minutes.
4. Remove cake from oven and allow to cool completely.
5. In a large bowl, beat remaining heavy whipping cream, cocoa powder, and erythritol until smooth.
6. Spread the cream on the cake evenly.

7. Place cake in the refrigerator for 30 minutes.
8. Slice and serve.

Per Serving: Net Carbs: 5g; Calories: 282 Total Fat: 26.1g; Saturated Fat: 15.6g

Protein: 7.1g; Carbs: 10.1g; Fiber: 5.1g; Sugar: 0.9g; Fat 83% / Protein 10% / Carbs 7%

Fudgy Chocolate Cake

Serves: 12

Preparation time: 10 minutes Cooking time: 30 minutes

Ingredients:

- 6 eggs
- 1 ½ cup erythritol
- ½ cup almond flour
- oz butter, melted
- oz unsweetened chocolate, melted
- Pinch of salt

Directions:

1. Preheat the oven to 350 F/ 180 C.
2. Grease 8-inch spring-form cake pan with butter and set aside.
3. In a large bowl, beat eggs until foamy.
4. Add sweetener and stir well.
5. Add melted butter, chocolate, almond flour, and salt and stir until combined.
6. Pour batter in the prepared cake pan and bake in preheated oven for 30 minutes.
7. Remove cake from oven and allow to cool completely.
8. Slice and serve.

Per Serving: Net Carbs: 4g; Calories: 360; Total Fat: 37.6g; Saturated Fat: 21.6g

Protein: 7.2g; Carbs: 8.6g; Fiber: 4.6g; Sugar: 0.6g; Fat 90% / Protein 7% / Carbs 3%

Cinnamon Almond Cake

Serves: 6

Preparation time: 10 minutes Cooking time: 20 minutes

Ingredients:

- 4 eggs
- 1 tsp orange zest
- 2/3 cup dried cranberries
- 1 ½ cups almond flour
- 1 tsp vanilla extract
- 2 tsp mixed spice
- 2 tsp cinnamon
- ¼ cup erythritol
- 1 cup butter, softened

Directions:

1. Preheat the oven to 350 F/ 180 C.
2. In a bowl, add sweetener and melted butter and beat until fluffy.
3. Add cinnamon, vanilla, and mixed spice and stir well.
4. Add egg one by one and stir until well combined.
5. Add almond flour, orange zest, and cranberries and mix until well combined.
6. Pour batter in a greased cake pan and bake in preheated oven for 20 minutes.

7. Slice and serve.

Per Serving: Net Carbs: 4.3g; Calories: 484; Total Fat: 47.6g; Saturated Fat: 21.3g

Protein: 10g; Carbs: 8.2g; Fiber: 3.9g; Sugar: 1.8g; Fat 88% / Protein 8% / Carbs 4%

Intermediate: Lemon Cake

Serves: 10

Preparation time: 10 minutes Cooking time: 60 minutes

Ingredients:

- 4 eggs
- 2 tbsp lemon zest
- ½ cup fresh lemon juice
- ¼ cup erythritol
- 1 tbsp vanilla
- ½ cup butter softened
- 2 tsp baking powder
- ¼ cup coconut flour
- 2 cups almond flour

Directions:

1. Preheat the oven to 300 F/ 150 C.
2. Grease 9-inch loaf pan with butter and set aside.
3. In a large bowl, whisk all ingredients until a smooth batter is formed.
4. Pour batter into the loaf pan and bake in preheated oven for 60 minutes.
5. Slice and serve.

Per Serving: Net Carbs: 3.6g; Calories: 244; Total Fat: 22.3g; Saturated Fat: 7.3g Protein: 7.3g; Carbs: 6.3g; Fiber: 2.7g; Sugar: 1.5g; Fat 83% / Protein 12% / Carbs 5%

CANDY: BEGINNER

Strawberry Candy

Serves: 12

Preparation time: 10 minutes Cooking time: 10 minutes

Ingredients:

- 3 fresh strawberries
- 1/2 cup butter, softened
- 8 oz cream cheese, softened
- 1/2 tsp vanilla
- 3/4 cup Swerve

Directions:

1. Add all ingredients into the food processor and process until smooth.
2. Pour mixture into the silicone candy mold and place in the refrigerator for 2 hours or until candy is hardened.
3. Serve and enjoy.

Per Serving: Net Carbs: 0.8g; Calories: 136 Total Fat: 14.3g; Saturated Fat: 9g

Protein: 1.5g; Carbs: 0.9g; Fiber: 0.1g; Sugar: 0.2g; Fat 94% / Protein 4% / Carbs 2%

Blackberry Candy

Serves: 8

Preparation time: 5 minutes Cooking time: 5 minutes

Ingredients:

- 1/2 cup fresh blackberries
- 1/4 cup cashew butter
- 1 tbsp fresh lemon juice
- 1/2 cup coconut oil
- 1/2 cup unsweetened coconut milk

Directions:

1. Heat cashew butter, coconut oil, and coconut milk in a pan over medium- low heat, until just warm.
2. Transfer cashew butter mixture to the blender along with remaining ingredients and blend until smooth.
3. Pour mixture into the silicone candy mold and refrigerate until set.
4. Serve and enjoy.

Per Serving: Net Carbs: 2.9g; Calories: 203; Total Fat: 21.2g; Saturated Fat: 15.8g

Protein: 1.9g; Carbs: 3.9g; Fiber: 1g; Sugar: 1g; Fat 92% / Protein 3% / Carbs 5%

COOKIES: BEGINNER

Almond Butter Cookies

Serves: 10

Preparation time: 5 minutes Cooking time: 10 minutes

Ingredients:

- 1 cup almond flour
- 1 tsp vanilla
- ¼ cup erythritol
- ¼ cup butter softened
- Pinch of salt

Directions:

1. Preheat the oven to 350 F/ 180 C.
2. Line baking tray with parchment paper and set aside.
3. Add all ingredients into the food processor and process until dough is formed, about 2 minutes.
4. Make cookies from dough and place on a prepared baking tray.
5. Bake in preheated oven for 10 minutes.
6. Remove cookies from oven and allow to cool completely.
7. Serve and enjoy.

Per Serving: Net Carbs: 1.3g; Calories: 106; Total Fat: 10.2g; Saturated Fat: 3.3g Protein: 2.5g; Carbs: 2.5g; Fiber: 1.2g; Sugar: 0.5g; Fat 86% / Protein 10% / Carbs 4%

Crunchy Shortbread Cookies

Serves: 6

Preparation time: 10 minutes Cooking time: 10 minutes

Ingredients:

- 1 ¼ cup almond flour
- ½ tsp vanilla
- 3 tbsp butter, softened
- ¼ cup Swerve
- Pinch of salt

Directions:

1. Preheat the oven to 350 F/ 180 C.
2. In a bowl, mix together almond flour, swerve, and salt.
3. Add vanilla and butter and mix until dough is formed.
4. Make cookies from mixture and place on a baking tray.
5. Bake in preheated oven for 10 minutes.
6. Allow to cool completely then serve.

Per Serving: Net Carbs: 2.6g; Calories: 185; Total Fat: 17.4g; Saturated Fat: 4.5g

Protein: 5.1g; Carbs: 5.1g; Fiber: 2.5g; Sugar: 0.9g; Fat 84% / Protein 11% / Carbs 5%

FROZEN DESSERT: BEGINNER

Raspberry Yogurt

Serves: 6

Preparation time: 10 minutes Cooking time: 10 minutes

Ingredients:

- 2 cups plain yogurt
- 5 oz fresh raspberries
- ½ cup erythritol

Directions:

1. Add all ingredients into the blender and blend until smooth.
2. Transfer blended mixture in air-tight container and place in the refrigerator for 40 minutes.
3. Remove yogurt mixture from refrigerator and blend again until smooth.
4. Pour in container and place in the refrigerator for 30 minutes.
5. Serve and enjoy.

Per Serving: Net Carbs: 7g; Calories: 70 Total Fat: 1.9g; Saturated Fat: 0.8g Protein: 5.1g; Carbs: 8.5g; Fiber: 1.5g; Sugar: 6.8g; Fat 26% / Protein 32% / Carbs 42%

Coconut Butter Popsicle

Serves: 12

Preparation time: 5 minutes Cooking time: 5 minutes

Ingredients:

- 2 cans unsweetened coconut milk
- 1 tsp liquid stevia
- 1/2 cup peanut butter

Directions:

1. Add all ingredients into the blender and blend until smooth.
2. Pour mixture into the molds and place in the refrigerator for 3 hours or until set.
3. Serve and enjoy.

Per Serving: Net Carbs: 3.1g; Calories: 175 Total Fat: 17.4g; Saturated Fat: 10.7g

Protein: 3.5g; Carbs: 3.7g; Fiber: 0.6g; Sugar: 2.6g; Fat 87% / Protein 7% / Carbs 6%

Raspberry Sorbet

Serves: 5

Preparation time: 10 minutes Cooking time: 10 minutes

Ingredients:

- 2 1/2 cups fresh raspberries
- 1 tbsp fresh lemon juice
- 1/3 cup erythritol
- 1/3 cup unsweetened coconut milk
- 1 tsp liquid stevia
- Pinch of sea salt

Directions:

1. Add all ingredients into the blender and blend until smooth.
2. Transfer blended mixture into the container and place in the refrigerator for 20 minutes.
3. After 20 minutes pour sorbet mixture into the ice cream maker and churn according to the machine instructions.
4. Pour into the air-tight container and place in the refrigerator for 1-2 hours.
5. Serve chilled and enjoy.

Per Serving: Net Carbs: 4g; Calories: 41; Total Fat: 1.9g; Saturated Fat: 0.7g

Protein: 1g; Carbs: 8g; Fiber: 4g; Sugar: 2.8g; Fat 45% / Protein 10% / Carbs 45%

Strawberry Yogurt

Serves: 8

Preparation time: 5 minutes Cooking time: 5 minutes

Ingredients:

- 4 cups frozen strawberries
- 1/2 cup plain yogurt
- 1 tsp liquid stevia
- 1 tbsp fresh lemon juice

Directions:

1. Add all ingredients into the blender and blend until yogurt is smooth and creamy.
2. Serve immediately and enjoy.

Per Serving: Net Carbs: 6.1g; Calories: 36; Total Fat: 0.9g; Saturated Fat: 0.2g

Protein: 1g; Carbs: 7.6g; Fiber: 1.5g; Sugar: 5.6g; Fat 22% / Protein 11% / Carbs 67%

BREAKFAST RECIPES

Beginners: Simmered Garlic Bread

All out: 1 hr. 20 min

Prep: 10 min

Cook: 1 hr. 10 min

Yield: 6 to 8 servings

Nutritional Values:

Fat: 35 g.

Protein: 6 g.

Carbs: 5 g.

Ingredients

- 4 heads garlic
- 1/3 cup extra-virgin olive oil
- 3 sprigs thyme, in addition to 1 tablespoon finely slashed
- Dark salt and crisply ground dark pepper
- 8 tablespoons unsalted margarine (1 stick), at room temperature
- 1 portion of good, hard bread, cut into cuts

Direction
1. Preheat broiler to 350 degrees F.
2. Cut top from each head of garlic, uncovering the cloves. Spot heads of garlic (cut side up), on a bit of rock solid aluminum foil. Pour olive oil over them, and top with thyme springs. Season with salt and pepper. Wrap the foil firmly. Spot in a little ovenproof container, and heat until the cloves start to fly out, around 60 minutes. Expel from the stove and cool.
3. To expel the cloves, open the foil and crush the lower some portion of the head of garlic. In a little bowl, squash the cloves to frame a glue. (Now the glue can be utilized or put away in the

   cooler or cooler.)
4. Add margarine and slashed thyme to the bowl, mixing to join. Season with salt and pepper, to taste.
5. Toast the two sides of the bread, utilizing a hot barbecue, flame broil dish, or grill. Spread the cooked garlic margarine glue onto the toasted bread. Serve right away.

Basil Pesto Bread

Complete: 15 min

Prep: 10 min

Cook: 5 min

Yield: 6 servings

Nutritional Values:

Fat: 27 g.

Protein: 4 g.

Carbs: 3 g.

Ingredients

- 2 cups new basil leaves
- 1/2 cup ground Parmesan or Romano
- 1/2 cup pine nuts, toasted
- 4 garlic cloves, generally hacked
- 1/4 teaspoon salt
- 1/2 cup olive oil
- 1 loaf

Direction

1. For the pesto, consolidate all fixings in a nourishment processor or blender. Puree until the blend shapes a smooth, thick glue. Cut the loaf the long way on a level plane. Spread the pesto over the cut sides of the loaf and toast in the broiler until fresh and brilliant.

Broken Black Pepper Bread

Complete: 4 hr 45 min

Prep: 4 hr

Cook: 45 min

Yield: 1 portion bread

Nutritional Values:

Calories: 34, Total Fat: 5.1 g, Saturated Fat: 0.3 g, Carbs: 1.5 g, Sugars: 0.3 g, Protein: 1.3 g

Ingredients

- 2 cups in addition to 2 tablespoons milk
- 3 tablespoons unsalted spread
- 2 tablespoons sugar
- 1/2 teaspoons butcher's crush broke dark pepper
- One 1/4-ounce bundle dynamic dry yeast
- 5 cups generally useful flour
- 1 tablespoon fine salt
- Vegetable oil, as required

Direction

2. In a little pot, consolidate the milk, spread, sugar, and pepper. Spot over medium-high warmth and achieve to 110 degrees F. Expel from the warmth and sprinkle the yeast over the outside of the milk. Put aside until frothy, around 10 minutes.
3. In the mean time, in an enormous bowl, whisk together the flour and salt.

4. Pour the milk and yeast blend into the bowl of flour and blend until a delicate, battered blend is shaped. Move the blend to a well-floured work surface and ply until a delicate versatile batter is framed, around 10 minutes. Move the mixture to a softly oiled bowl, spread with a kitchen towel, and spot in a warm spot, until puffed and multiplied in size, around 2 hours.
5. Spot a rack in the focal point of the broiler and preheat to 400 degrees F. Move the mixture to the work surface and, utilizing your hands, delicately straighten it into a 10-inch-long oval shape. Crease the batter into thirds longwise, covering the sides in the inside. Press down on the covering sides to seal and make a crease. Spot it crease side-down in a buttered 9 by 5- inch portion dish, spread with a kitchen towel, and come back to the hottest piece of the kitchen until the mixture has ascended around 1/2 crawls over the highest point of the container, around 1/2 to 2 hours.
6. Brush the highest point of the batter gently with warm water and, utilizing a sharp blade, make 1/4-inch-profound cut down the middle. Prepare until brilliant darker, around 30 minutes.
7. Expel the portion from the skillet and spot in the focal point of the rack. Keep heating until the portion sounds empty when riveted gently with your knuckles on the base and top, and a thermometer embedded in the inside peruses 200 degrees F., around 15 minutes.
8. Move the bread portion to a cooling rack and let cool for 2 hours before utilizing.

Pennsylvania Dutch Potato and Bread Filling

Preparation Time: 2 hours Servings:8

Nutritional Values:

Fat: 37 g.

Protein: 5 g.

Carbs: 5 g.

Ingredients

- 6 huge potatoes, cut in pieces
- 2 medium onions, cleaved
- 6 stalks celery, cleaved little
- Enough vegetable oil for saute

- 8-10 bits of old bread, broken into scaled down pieces
- 1/4 to 1/2 cup milk
- 4 crude eggs, beaten
- Salt and pepper
- Salt and pepper
- 4-5 tablespoons new parsley, hacked fine
- 1-2 tablespoons poultry flavoring
- Stock from the giblets and neck
- Stock from the giblets and neck
- 1/2 stick of spread, cut into pieces

Direction

1. Dampen bread with milk. Crush the potatoes in an enormous bowl. (I utilize a little cooking skillet, and after that I broil the filling directly in it.) Add every other fixing including all flavors and oil from saute. When including the eggs, include a tad bit of the hot blend to the eggs first and beat well, in order to not scramble them when they go into the entire blend.
2. Blend completely. On the off chance that it needs more dampness, include the stock, a little at any given moment. Taste to ensure enough flavors are included. Include progressively salt and pepper and poultry flavoring, if necessary.
3. Heat at 350 degrees in a lubed goulash dish or broiling container until extremely hot and seared, normally 60 minutes. Speck the top with taps of spread before putting into broiler. I realize a few people slash the giblets and add to the filling, yet I don't.

LUNCH RECIPES

Beginners: Low-Carb Cream Cheese Rolls

Servings: 6 rolls

Nutritional Values:

Calorie 0.8 g Net Carbs ; 4.2 g Proteins; 8 g Fat; 91.3 Calories

Ingredients:

- Large eggs – 3
- Full-fat cream cheese - cubed & cold – 3 oz.
- Cream of tartar - .125 tsp.
- Salt - .125 tsp.

Directions:
1. Warm up the oven to 300°F. Line a baking tin with parchment paper. Spritz the pan with cooking oil spray.
2. The yolks should separated from the eggs and place the whites in a non- greasy container. Whisk with the tartar until stiff.
3. In another container, whisk the cream cheese, salt, and yolks until smooth.
4. Fold in the whites of the eggs, mixing well using a spatula. Mound a scoop of whites over the yolk mixture and fold together as you rotate the dish. Continue the process until well combined. The process helps to eliminate the air bubbles.
5. Portion six large spoons of the mixture onto the prepared pan. Mash the tops with the spatulate to slightly flatten.
6. Bake until browned (30-40 min.).
7. Cool a few minutes in the pan. Then, carefully arrange them on a wire rack to cool.
8. Store in a zipper-type bag – open slightly – and store in the fridge for a

   couple of days for best results.

Homemade Sesame Breadsticks

Nutritional Values:

Calories: 53.6, Total Fat: 5 g, Saturated Fat: 1.6 g, Carbs: 1.1 g, Sugars: 0.2 g, Protein: 1.6 g

Serves: 5 breadsticks

Ingredients:

- 1 Egg White
- 2 Tbsp Almond Flour
- 1 tsp Himalayan Pink Salt
- 1 Tbsp Extra Virgin Olive Oil
- ½ tsp Sesame Seeds

Directions:

1. Preheat your oven to 320F / 160C. Set aside after parchment paper is lined with the baking sheet.
2. Whisk the egg white and add the flour as well as half each the salt and olive oil.
3. Knead until you get smooth dough, divide into 5 pieces and roll into breadsticks.
4. Place on the prepared sheet, brush with the remaining olive oil, place the shee and sprinkle with the sesame seeds and the remaining salt.
5. Bake for about 20 minutes. Allow to cool slightly before serving.

Herb Bread

Nutritional Values:

Calories: 421, Total Fat: 37.4 g, Saturated Fat: 14.8 g, Carbs: 9.4 g, Sugars: 0.9 g, Protein: 15.1 g Serves: 4

Ingredients:

- 2 Tbsp Coconut Flour
- 1 ½ cups Almond Flour
- 2 Tbsp Fresh Herbs of choice, chopped
- 2 Tbsp Ground Flax Seeds
- 1 ½ tsp Baking Soda
- ¼ tsp Salt
- 5 Eggs
- 1 Tbsp Apple Cider Vinegar
- ¼ cup Coconut Oil, melted

Directions:

1. Preheat your oven to 350F / 175C. Grease a loaf pan and set aside.
2. Add the coconut flour, almond flour, herbs, flax, baking soda, and salt to your food processor. Pulse to combine and then add the eggs, vinegar, and oil.
3. Transfer the batter to the prepared loaf pan and bake in the preheated oven for about half an hour.
4. Once baked and golden brown, remove from the oven, set aside to cool, slice and eat.

Almond Keto Bread

Nutritional Values:

Calories: 302, Total Fat: 28.6 g, Saturated Fat: 3 g, Carbs: 7.3g, Sugars: 1.2 g, Protein: 8.5 g Serves: 10 slices

Ingredients:

- 3 cups Almond Flour
- 1 tsp Baking Soda
- 2 tsp Baking Powder
- ¼ tsp Salt
- ¼ cup Almond Milk
- ½ cup + 2 Tbsp Olive Oil
- 3 Eggs

Directions:

1. Preheat your oven to 300F / 149C. Grease a loaf pan (e.g. 9x5) and set aside.
2. Combine all the ingredients and transfer the batter to the prepared loaf pan.
3. Bake in the preheated oven for an hour.
4. Once baked, remove from the oven, allow to cool, slice and eat.

SNACKS RECIPES

Beginners: Bread with zucchini and walnuts

Servings: 12

Cooking time: 85 minutes

Nutrients per one serving: Calories: 123 | Fats: 15.3 g | Carbs: 4.8 g | Proteins: 6.6 g

Ingredients:

- 1 cup almond flour
- 1 zucchini
- 3 eggs
- 1 tbsp erythritol
- 2 tbsp walnuts
- 3 tbsp olive oil
- 1 tsp vanilla
- 1 tsp baking powder
- 1 tsp cinnamon
- ½ tsp ginger powder
- A pinch of salt

Cooking process:
1. The oven to be preheated to 180°C (356°F).
2. In a bowl, mix the eggs, butter, and vanilla. In another container, mix the flour, sweetener, baking powder, cinnamon, ginger powder, and salt.
3. Chop the zucchini until uniformity. Drain excess liquid.
4. Add the dry ingredients and zucchini to the egg. Beat them by a mixer for 1 minute until uniformity.
5. Lay out the dough into the greased form. Decorate with chopped walnuts.

Garlic bread

Servings: 10

Cooking time: 20 minutes

Nutrients per one serving:

Calories: 80 | Fats: 15 g | Carbs: 1.6 g | Proteins: 9 g

Ingredients:

- 1 package bread baking mass
- 1 ⅓ cup warm water
- 1 tbsp butter
- 3 garlic cloves
- 1 tbsp dry oregano

Cooking process:

1. In a bowl, mix the dough from the bread baking mass and water. Make a long baguette.
2. Cover the baking sheet with parchment. Place the baguette on the baking sheet and make shallow notches.
3. Bake in the oven at a temperature of 180°C (356°F) for 25 minutes.
4. Prepare the garlic butter. Mix the butter, chopped garlic, and oregano.
5. Grate hot bread with garlic butter and send to the oven for 10 minutes.

Sesame bread

Servings: 3

Cooking time: 20 minutes

Nutrients per one serving:

Calories: 82 | Fats: 12 g | Carbs: 1 g | Proteins: 7 g

Ingredients:

- 5 tbsp sesame flour
- 1 egg
- 1 tbsp butter
- ½ tsp baking powder
- A pinch of salt

Cooking process:

1. Mix the ingredients.
2. Melt the butter to room temperature.

Add butter and egg to the mass, mix well.

3. Pour the dough into a baking dish and bake in the oven at 180°C (356°F) for 15 minutes.

Focaccia

Servings: 2-4

Cooking time: 35 minutes

Nutrients per one serving:

Calories: 78 | Fats: 10 g | Carbs: 5 g | Proteins: 8 g

Ingredients:

- 1 package bread baking mass
- 1 ⅓ cup water
- 2 tbsp olive oil
- ¼ cup olives
- ½ tsp sea salt
- 1 tsp dry rosemary

Cooking process:

1. Mix the dough from the bread mass, water, and olive oil.
2. Cover the baking sheet with parchment.
3. Roll out the dough on a baking into a flat cake. Decorate with olives, sprinkle with salt and rosemary.
4. Bake in the oven at 200°C (400°F) for 20 minutes.
5. Important! You can use dried tomatoes, cheese, bacon, garlic, and mushrooms as a decorating.

THE KETO LUNCH

In this chapter, we'll provide a seven-day menu that you can use for some easy to make but extremely delicious keto lunches.

Monday: Lunch: Keto Meatballs

Make these ahead of time because these delicious meatballs are freezable. Take a few to work along with some sugar-free marinara sauce and zoodles (zucchini noodles) for a delicious keto lunch.

Variation tip: change the seasonings to make different flavors, like taco or barbecue.

Prep Time: 5 minutes Cook Time: 18 minutes

Servings: 4

What's in it

- Grass-fed ground beef (1 pound)
- Chopped fresh parsley (1.5 t)
- Onion powder (.75 t)
- Garlic powder (.75 t)
- Kosher salt (.75 t)
- Fresh ground black pepper (.5 t)

How it's made

1. Turn oven to 400-degrees F to preheat.
2. Using parchment paper, line a baking sheet.
3. Put beef into a medium-sized glass bowl with other ingredients

and mix with hands until just combined. Avoid over-mixing as this will result in tough meatballs.
4. Roll into 8 meatballs and place on the lined baking sheet.
5. Bake for 15-18 minutes until done all the way through.

Net carbs: 3 grams Fat: 17 grams

Protein: 11 grams

Sugars: 2 grams

Tuesday: Lunch: Mason Jar Salad

So colorful and full of flavor. This salad is portable. Use any vegetable you have on hand.

Variation tip: try different kinds of protein, cheese or seeds.

Prep Time: 10 minutes Cook Time: None

Servings: 1

What's in it

- Cooked, diced chicken (4 ounces)
- Baby spinach (1/6 ounce)
- Cherry tomatoes (1/6 ounce)
- Bell pepper (1/6 ounce)
- Cucumber (1/6 ounce)
- Green onion (1/2 qty)
- Extra virgin olive oil (4 T)

How it's made

1. Chop vegetables.
2. Stuff spinach at the bottom of jar.
3. Layer the rest of the vegetables.
4. Keep olive oil in a separate container until ready to eat.

Net carbs: 4 grams Fat: 55 grams

Protein: 71 grams

Sugars: 1 gram

Wednesday: Lunch: The Smoked Salmon Special

This may be the easiest lunch special ever.

Flavorful, smoky, pink salmon poses on your

plate next to dark, green spinach as a feast for the eyes and the body.

Variation tip: serve with arugula or cabbage. Prep Time: 5 minutes

Cook Time: None Serves 2

What's in it

- Wild caught smoked salmon (.5 ounces)
- Mayonnaise (generous dollop)
- Baby spinach (large handful)
- Extra virgin olive oil (.5 T)
- Lime wedge (1 qty)
- Kosher salt (to taste)
- Fresh ground pepper (to taste)

How it's made

1. Place salmon (or any fatty fish like sardines or mackerel) and spinach on a plate.
2. Add a large spoonful of mayonnaise and the lime wedge.
3. Drizzle oil atop the baby spinach (or try arugula or cabbage shredded as if for slaw)
4. Sprinkle with a little salt and pepper. Net carbs: None

Fat: 109 grams

Protein: 105 grams Sugars: None

KETO AT DINNER

Monday: Dinner: Beef short ribs in a slow cooker

With a little prep, you will have a hot meal waiting for you at the end of a long day.

Variation tip: serve over diced cauliflower or with celery.

Prep Time: 15 minutes Cook Time: 4 hours

Servings: 4

What's in it

- Boneless short ribs or bone-in (2 pounds)
- Kosher salt (to taste)
- Fresh ground pepper (to taste)
- Extra virgin olive oil (2 T)
- Chopped white onion (1 qty)
- Garlic (3 cloves)
- Bone broth (1 cup)
- Coconut aminos (2 T)
- Tomato paste (2 T)
- Red wine (1.5 cups)

How it's made
1. In a large skillet over medium heat, add olive oil. Season meat with salt and pepper. Brown both sides.
2. Add broth and browned ribs to slow cooker
3. Put remaining ingredients into the skillet.
4. Bring to a boil and cook until onions are tender. About 5 minutes.
5. Pour over ribs.
6. Set to 4 to 6 hours on high or 8 to 10 hours on low.

Net carbs: 1 gram

Fat: 63 grams

Protein: 24 grams

Sugars: 1 gram

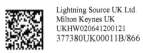
Lightning Source UK Ltd.
Milton Keynes UK
UKHW020641200121
377380UK00011B/866